Daily Habit Makeover

Beat Procrastination,

Get More Productive,

Focus Better,

And Become Healthier in Body and Mind

By Zoe McKey

Communication Coach and Social Development Trainer

zoemckey@gmail.com

www.zoemckey.com

rendering medical, legal or other professional advice or services. If professional assistance is required, the services of a competent professional person should be sought. The author shall not be liable for damages arising herefrom. The fact that an individual, organization of website is referred to in this work as a citation and/or potential source of further information does not mean that the author endorses the information the individual, organization to website may provide or recommendations they/it may make. Further, readers should be aware that Internet websites listed in this work might have changed or disappeared between when this work was written and when it is read.

For general information on the products and services or to obtain technical support, please contact the author.

Thank you for choosing my book! I would like to show my appreciation for the trust you gave me by giving **FREE GIFTS** for you!

For more information visit www.zoemckey.com

The checklist talks about *5 key elements of building self-confidence* and contains extra actionable worksheets with practice exercises for deeper learning.

Learn how to:

- Solve 80% of you self-esteem issues with one simple change
- Keep your confidence permanent without falling back to self-doubt
- Not fall into the trap of promising words
- Overcome anxiety
- Be confident among other people

The cheat sheet teaches you three key daily routine techniques to become more productive, have less stress in your life, and be more well-balanced. It also has a step-by-step sample sheet that you can fill in with your daily routines.

Discover how to:

- Overcome procrastination following 8 simple steps
- Become more organized
- Design your yearly, monthly, weekly and daily tasks in the most productive way.
- 3 easy tricks to level up your mornings

Table Of Contents

Prologue

This book starts where everything ended. You died. (Pretty morbid start.) You look at your grave and your weeping family. Your tombstone says, "Here lies (your name), who lived 80 years." Rain starts to pour, and your friends and family slowly go home.

You have nothing else to do but contemplate your life. You can do it honestly now. You've passed the point of no return. It's game over. Nothing bad can happen if you admit what you should or shouldn't have done in those 80 years.

Ask yourself: *Was I truly happy? Did I do everything I wanted? Do I have regrets about my life? If I could go back, would I say yes to any opportunities I missed? Or no to some I accepted? Would I be more active, procrastinate less, and enjoy more of life's gifts?*

If you feel you have no regrets, you did everything you wanted, and there's nothing you'd do differently, you are one of the few who lived a full and happy life.

However, if you feel you missed out on some chances, that you would have liked more achievement in your life, or that you said no too many times, this book can help you.

People don't realize they've missed opportunities until is too late. There are some sayings like: "I'd rather apologize than ask permission," and "It's better to regret what you have done than what you haven't." (Paul Arden) I think there is truth to these statements.

What do you think went wrong? Did you say no to many possibilities? Did you feel you didn't have any opportunities at all? Did you try to create any? You had opportunities and wishes and dreams, but did you just not ever have the time, money, and energy for them?

All the answers to the lack of fulfillment in our lives can be found somewhere in your bad daily routines. If you have a clear priority list, well-defined goals, and a reasonable, healthy daily schedule for them, you can find the time, energy, even the money to say yes more and enjoy your life to the fullest!

I was joking. You're not dead. Not at all. You are very alive, here in this moment, and you have many more decades until you contemplate your life from the grave. Just don't forget that day will come and every day it comes closer. This is the beauty of life — it's limited. You can never know when your last day will be. You'll never be younger or more beautiful than you are right now. You'll never have this moment again. You have time, but none to be wasted.

So don't waste it with regrets and complaints. That's behind you. You didn't sign up to be a cheerleader in high school? You won't be able to rewrite it. Did you choose to be an actress instead of a doctor? There's no point in thinking, *If I had done it differently, then...* or *If I had married Dr. Schultz instead of this sad sack...* That's the past. It resulted in your present, that's true. But your present forms what is ahead of you.

How can you make your future better? By changing the things that led you to a dissatisfied present.

Life isn't very complicated, as far as the big picture goes. Our days are mostly repetitive — composed of routines. What we see on social media — the special moments, the highs, the giant Nutella pancakes and holidays at Bali — are just blinks of an eye, heightened moments of an otherwise normal life. Everybody's life is composed of routines, most of the time. This is why it is so important to have good routines. Good routines help you get to those occasional highs that make life special. Also, good routines are the ones that keep regrets out of your life.

All the distractions and barriers that stand between you and your ability to build healthy routines should be removed. The biggest roadblock usually is procrastination. The "oh, I will do it tomorrow" mentality seems harmless, but in fact, it can do a lot of damage if you don't focus on overcoming it. The first part of the book will talk about procrastination — its causes, its types — and provide a detailed action plan for how to overcome it.

The second part of the book will give you a broad perspective on how to organize your day to be more productive. It will also cover how you can keep up your productivity, best practices to bring out the most in each day, and advice from the world's top entrepreneurs.

The third part of the book will discuss daily philosophies you can wrap your mindset around. Having a coherent philosophy for life can make you more accepting of death, among other things. Acknowledging the inevitability of death will also highlight what in life is worth fighting for. Those who live without the core values of life will desperately try to delay their deaths, because their improvised or "trend oriented" values convinced them they were on the right track and that they had time. People who think they will live forever are more likely to waste their lives than those who understand that human life is perishable and our days are numbered.

Chapter 1: Procrastination

The first part of this book discusses one of the greatest obstacles in the way of a good life: procrastination. This seemingly harmless habit can pretty much leave you on your deathbed with a life full of regrets.

Procrastination, if not done in excess, is a natural state of mind. There's nothing wrong with you; everybody does it. If somebody tells you that he or she doesn't procrastinate, it's a lie. In small doses, it can be even helpful. If you don't take a pause from time to time, you can burn out very quickly. But there's a level above which procrastination prevents you from taking action, moving forward, and living a quality life. You know, the more you do, the better you feel. In the following pages, I present the dark side of procrastination. If you can relate to any or many of the descriptions, think about how much your life would improve if you changed it.

The Psychology Of Procrastination

Maybe tomorrow... Today is yesterday's tomorrow.

Procrastination slows development, derails your progress toward your goals, and replaces action with anger and despair. It is the gravedigger of success. The difference between success and failure is action. Procrastination is a highly motivated state. We are motivated to do nothing, to avoid difficulties, obstacles, and emotionally intolerable situations.

"Motivation is what gets you started. Habit is what keeps you going." — Jim Rohn.

A story on procrastination:

Rachel knew she had to finish her assignment at the end of the month, but it was only the seventh. She knew she had a lot of time left. She was confident in her abilities and knew that she'd be able to finish the work in one week — worst case. So she didn't do anything for two weeks. As each day passed, she convinced herself more and more that she had time. Each day, she had to come up with better explanations and justifications.

When there was only a week left until the deadline, she rationalized that six days should also be enough for her to finish if she worked hard and stayed up late. When only six days were left, something unpredictable happened, so she couldn't start working. The next day, she finally sat down and started doing research about the assignment. It turned out that she vastly underestimated the time required. The scarcity of time made her anxious, so she couldn't work as focused as she knew she could.

One day before the deadline, she still had 30% of the work left, so she quickly patched up the rest of her assignment to meet the deadline. The assignment wasn't rejected, but it wasn't given a top mark, either.

If she had started doing the assignment on time, she could have done an outstanding job. If she dedicated the first week to it instead of the last, she could have finished it in one week as she estimated because stress and time scarcity wouldn't have invaded her brain. But who has ever done such a thing in the history of humanity? Do something in the first week instead of the last?

Often, we know what to do, and why and how we should do it. We just haven't gotten to that unpleasant time when we absolutely must do it. Many people work this way. If there is no coercive force, they sit and pass the time because it is easiest, most convenient, and requires the least amount of effort.

Let's say you have a task to do, and you realize you are just putting it off. Right after the realization, start taking action immediately. Do something small. It doesn't even have to be directly connected to the task you're delaying. Just do something that makes you happy, that you enjoy, and which makes you feel motivated. After that, you might find it easier to return to the basic task and take steps to solving the problem.

It is easier to have continuous momentum than it is to get up to speed, go full force, then come to a stop, then go full force again, and then relax. These ups and downs really only work during high-intensity cardio trainings. When we talk about good routines, constant starts and pauses sap your energy and enthusiasm and cloud your motivation.

If you are constantly in motion, making decisions and doing things, you get into a flow state of mind. This doesn't mean you burn your candle on both ends and suffer a heart attack at the age of 35. It just means you routinely condition your mindset to take action and ditch procrastination. It will be a lot easier to get started on assignments in time, if you don't have to waste extra energy with self-nagging.

Toddlers don't procrastinate. When they are hungry or thirsty, they let you know right away, sometimes quite forcefully. No waiting or procrastinating in their agenda. They start crying. They need their diaper changed right now, not tomorrow or the next month.

But then they start learning from their surroundings. About 70-75% of young people —

college-age to thirty or so —are procrastinators. Of older adults, about 25-30% are still in the procrastination trap, even though they've already experienced the downside of procrastination.

"My best friend is the one who brings out the best in me," Henry Ford stated at a reception.

Lara and Jack had been married for 12 years. They knew each other very well — knew each other's shortcomings and flaws. Lara knew that Jack was a passionate person who got fired up easily and jumped into execution very quickly. However, his motivation could decrease just as quickly. She knew that if his motivation hit rock bottom, he'd probably just stop working. She also knew that Jack could easily stay on track if he had to stop working before the most interesting task of the day. If he couldn't finish the big design, he'd be very eager to resume working the next day.

Jack knew how much trouble Lara went through to help him with his procrastinating habits. He considered himself very lucky for having such a woman by his side. After he finished each project, he found a way to show his gratitude and appreciation for her. Since Lara loved Jack's creative and unique surprises, she was almost looking forward to her husband's new projects so she could help him. They made a good team.

The weak wait for the opportunity; the strong make it happen. When we are awake, most of our actions are governed by our emotions; the result of our thoughts. We make decisions in our heads and are influenced by our conscious and subconscious minds.

The Reasons for Procrastination

Uncertainty, fear of failure (which people perceive as a threat), the inability to cope with certain things, subconscious fear — these are all reasons people procrastinate, and they depend on the person and situation.

The following list includes the main reasons people procrastinate. The first five are the most common reasons. The others are less frequently encountered; however, they round out the list to give you a more complete image.

1.) **Feeling overworked**. Things start to pile up. You don't even remember which task is most important. It is difficult to prioritize when there is too much to do. In your desperation, you start working on the task with the closest deadline. Sometimes you do things because they seem like easy fixes. This way, you can deceive yourself into feeling efficient.

2.) **Boring work.** Doing something you do not enjoy and don't see a way out of makes it hard to work. A task can be monotonous, tiresome, and make you sleepy. Doing the same thing day after day can get boring, if you cannot find something interesting that you like about it. People working in the same job for years often can't find motivation.

3.) **Fear.** Two related extremes of this feeling will lead to procrastination.

Fear of responsibility: When you stop procrastinating, you come face to face with an uncharted area of responsibility and that can scare you — for example, how many things you could have done while you were procrastinating — so you will start procrastinating again. Dare to face your flaws, to take the risk of error and failure. This is the only way to learn and move toward your dreams.

Fear of taking risks: This is a major barrier to personal development. Procrastinators see non-existent dangers in front of them, and their imagination exaggerates possible risks. There is no action without risk, and without action, there is no meaningful life. Obstacles litter the path to success.

4.) **Lack of motivation**. *"Why rush? It will have to get done sooner or later, but for now, it can wait."* It's not like you get an award for doing it. Some people may not like to upset the status quo. People who are subject to this type of procrastination prefer to do nothing unless it is certain that there is a reward for their action.

5.) **Shame**. In this case, you may feel it's embarrassing to ask for help. Shame can prevent you from asking for help when you need it.

6.) **Feeling paralyzed**. If the magnitude of the task is frightening, break the problem into smaller sub-steps and execute them. These smaller, easier parts will get you moving again. Accept that it won't be perfect the first time. How do you eat an elephant? One bite at a time.

7.) **Inability to analyze**. You are unable to see the forest for the trees. In other words, you can't decipher the task because of the details. It seems too big and complicated. What are you supposed to do? What is it about? Which way should you look at it? First things first, you need to know where to start, and then you can focus on the next step. And the next. At some point, the big picture becomes clearer. It's like approaching a destination while driving. First you may have to go through some rough or boring miles, and you may only be able to enjoy the view during the last leg of the journey.

8.) **Lack of priorities**. Those who do not list their tasks — in writing — according to their importance and urgency tend to jump from task to task. This can lead to chaos when they can't find the most important step to start their day, week, or month, and then choose to not do anything.

9.) **Forgetfulness.** You can get into the daily grind so deeply that you forget your basic task. That's how the brain protects itself from breaking a routine. You tend to turn on autopilot mode.

10.) **Nervousness.** We are afraid of personal confrontation and potential unpleasant criticism or failure. Inner tension manifests itself this way in almost everybody. There is a greater risk of making a mistake when you're nervous, and you want to avoid that. So you procrastinate. Being nervous, however, can be helpful because it mobilizes reserves, which can bring results.

11.) **Lethargy.** Sometimes people let their guards down and fall into self-pity. This is a sign of a lack of self-worth. They don't find themselves good or worthy enough to get off the couch.

12.) **Dependence.** Some people rely on others because they feel they can't do anything for themselves. They need somebody's approval or guidance. Without external control, they are like a ship without a captain, just drifting on the ocean.

13.) **Perfectionism.** These people obsessively strive for perfection. This type of procrastination can also be caused by a fear of failure and criticism. Often they tense up inside, their muscles stiffen, and their brains get foggy. They want to do their jobs without mistakes, and often they delay until "the moment of perfection" because they don't feel ready. This moment may never come.

14.) **Passing responsibility to others.** This person goofs and slacks off until someone else takes care of their work. They are in the background, pulling the strings until someone gets fed up and completes a large portion of their task.

15.) **Fatigue**. The excuse of fatigue is one of the best "excuse" methods. There is no human on earth who has not deferred something at least once because they were tired. The antidote is to rest. If you are truly worn out, then yes, it is a good excuse to delay things a bit. If you can't focus on your task, you won't be very productive anyway. Just make sure you are not making up this excuse because, as I said at the beginning, it's the best one, and you might end up believing it.

16.) **Over-commitment.** We take on more than we can handle. We want to play on many fields at once, and this leads to complete chaos. We take on so many burdens that we are crushed under the weight of them. Since it is hard to hold things together and figure out where to start, we tend to not do anything. This can make us seem unreliable and disorganized, even if we have the best intentions.

17.) **Lack of self-control**. Gaining awareness of our weaknesses and power to control them is maybe the most challenging task, especially if the consequences of not doing anything don't show up immediately. Learning how to control and motivate ourselves in moments of weakness is key to having a successful life.

18.) **Too many useless distractions**. Spending hours in front of the TV or computer is a nest for procrastination. The meaningless and empty programs, reports, and information that play on your emotions can lead you to postpone tasks.

Procrastination can be a short-term or long-term problem.

Short-term procrastination is when a project has a short deadline — for example, a cell phone bill that must be paid by the tenth. When the deadline is reached and the bill is paid, the bad feelings caused by procrastination are gone. After the deadline has passed and the problem gets solved, things get better, but in the meantime, tension and a feeling of stress and discomfort are considerably high.

Long-term procrastination is when someone procrastinates on a project that has no specific deadline. For example, if you decide to pursue self-employment, like starting a company, initially there is no deadline because nothing is started and nobody nags you to get things done. Other examples could be family troubles, living a healthy lifestyle, starting a relationship, or breaking up with somebody. With no deadline, motivational panic rarely occurs. There is no trigger. There is nothing to limit procrastination by reminding you of the consequences. It stretches and stretches until the end of time. Long-term procrastination produces hidden consequences.

Six Types of Procrastinators

1) The Avoider Procrastinator

The Avoider Procrastinators lack motivation to take any steps to change their situation. They are among those who give up their dreams for the benefit of others. They enrolled in college or started a training course because their parents or partner expected it. They don't say no because they avoid having to resist someone. They have jobs they don't like and don't find pleasure in. They are procrastinating on improving their own quality of life.

Avoider Procrastinators rely on others to choose directions and make decisions for them. On one hand, this is to avoid confrontation. On the other hand, they need agreement, approval, and guidance.

2) The Perfectionist Procrastinator

Perfectionist Procrastinators think that only perfection is good enough. They won't start working on a task until all the conditions are met and they have all the information they need to do the work. They document even the smallest details and collect everything they think they may need to complete an assignment.

They obsessively strive for perfection, which can be traced back to overbearing parents, a never-satisfied partner, fear of failure, and criticism. Often they tense up inside, and want to do their jobs without mistakes. They set the bar high. *"What would everyone say if I don't do a perfect job?"* They perceive making a mistake as shameful. Their dissatisfaction with themselves indicates a lack of self-confidence. Frequently, they overcomplicate things so much that the chance of running out of time increases.

If you want to defeat perfectionism, there are some critical questions you should think through. Take your tasks one at a time and examine each the following way:

a) Do I have all the necessary information to do the job? (Y/N)

b) Can I get the missing data/information to carry out the task before the deadline? (Y/N)

c) Am I able to finish the job as required by the deadline? (Y/N)

These questions are intended as a guide. You can write more questions, if that helps. They should have yes or no answers.

3) The Dreamer Procrastinator

Dreamer Procrastinators spend most of their days on autopilot mode. Often, they are so immersed in their own Wonderland that their actual job gets lost in the background. Sometimes they forget why they actually started what they were doing. They can dream interesting and colorful dreams, expand them, and fill these dreams with more details. There is no limit to their vivid imaginations.

They can design their jobs to be so beautiful and perfect in their Wonderland, but acting on the changes needed to make their dreams a reality hardly ever follows. When they feel the urge to start acting on something, their dream knight comes to aid them, saying, *"You still have time! You have to think it all through to have the big picture!"* That's how they delay action when they feel the pressure of time.

Dreamer Procrastinators mostly know what they want, they can make good plans, but at the moment of practical implementation, their whole system comes to a halt. They stop and postpone a certain job until tomorrow, or a vague "later." They become depressed; their mood darkens.

They are standing still, waiting, suffering until they can't take it, or until life hands them an alternative. Up until that moment, they are getting more frustrated. Suffering means they need to change something.

The potential is in you! You just need to learn to take advantage of it. You are a great planner! That's a good start. Your big task is to become a great implementer. It's no use having talents, skills, or knowledge, if you don't know how to use them. Every day, you should try a little harder to take action than you did the day before.

Walk the path you have chosen. Many start out on one path, but then stop and give up before they've finished. Many lose their faith, confidence, or endurance on the winding road. Say this out loud: **I will keep going**. Maybe success is waiting at the finish line just beyond the next turn.

4) The Negative Procrastinator

We were born to find our place in the world. Many people are waiting for the world to show them their place and where to go.

When things don't go the way Negative Procrastinators wanted, or when they get tasks that don't have an easy solution, suddenly, everything becomes dark. They see resistance and rejection everywhere.

Most people do most things the way they first learned them, repeating them almost automatically their whole lives, forging them into routines, and then habit. They get boxed in, and if they come across an unfamiliar situation, they come to a stop.

As long as people are in their comfort zones, it is hard to see the whole picture. Step out of your comfort zone. Every time negative thoughts pop up, immediately replace them with constructive, realistic ones and write them on a new page in that notebook you started to help you fight procrastination.

5) The Worrier Procrastinator

"Oh, what happens if...? What's going to happen? When will we do it?"

The Worrier Procrastinator sees the smallest hole in their path as a bottomless abyss. The slightest resistance or pushback scares him. He torments and tortures himself, postponing his task until the waves crash over his head.

This kind of procrastinator is stopped by the first negative opinion or circumstance, and will not move until they manage to calm down, convincing themselves that it was just a false alarm. And that may take a lot of time. Then another small cloud comes, and their worrying starts all over again.

Measure your abilities and limitations. Know your feelings and try to understand the reasons behind them. Rephrase your values so they work for you and not against you.

"Everything you want is on the other side of fear."
— Jack Canfield

Face your fears. Accept that they exist. Get to know your fears, and they will be much easier to live with and move on from. Once you start to understand your fear of responsibility and risk, it will be easier to manage these feelings. Everything depends on your point of view and attitude.

Experiencing fear is natural. This emotion is present in all of us. Your natural response toward fear can be twofold:

A. You can overcome your fears. You can use them as tools to be stronger and to reach your goals. Or...

B. You can let your fears gain control and hold you back from making your dreams come true.

Don't let the attitude in point B control you. Find a task where others have failed. Learning from their failures will help you succeed. If you follow these steps, you can find your greatest strength.

1. Ask yourself: What is the worst thing that can happen to me?
2. Write down the process and implications of this worst-case scenario as precisely as you can.
3. Prepare yourself mentally to accept it.
4. Write down every conceivable way to avoid the worst-case scenario.
5. Choose the solution you think is best.

Start working on the task. Just do it; finish it.

6) The Overachiever Procrastinator

The Overachiever Procrastinator is the person who takes on everything without thinking. They will do it all in their job and their social life, even if it's not possible. This is the person who works a lot and takes on even more — often other people's responsibilities — and things get chaotic.

As a result, the efficiency of their work is reduced and they get little done.

The space around them is not organized. They take on more than they can handle. The take on so much that, in the end, they collapse under the weight of it all. It is hard for them to manage things and figure out where to start. They are the ultimate "multitaskers."

If you are like this, you should develop the ability to focus on one particular thing at a time. Concentrate on one task and do it in the shortest time with the greatest efficiency. If you cannot focus on a task for an extended period, it will be difficult to be effective.

The Method of Overcoming Procrastination

In the process of discovering the law of nature, psychologists came up with a golden truth. The mind is capable of achieving anything you believe in. I'm not talking about education, degrees, or academics. Napoleon Hill was among the first who stated this fundamental law, which allows all of us to achieve our goals in a comprehensible form. He stated the following:

"Whatever the mind of man can conceive and believe, it can achieve."

Regardless of how many times you've failed in the past, you can make a difference now. You always can. The key is in your hands: *you must be willing to do it differently than before*. You may not achieve success, but at least you'll be closer to your goal. Remember Edison and his many experiments with the light bulb? Without him, maybe we'd still be using candles. Who knows what you could contribute to the world with resilience and grit? Maybe in 20 years, we'll sing hymns to you for being so persistent, brave, and smart.

There is a powerful force with no limits that is completely under your control. This force is greater than poverty and a lack of education, and greater than the sum of all your fears. With this force, you can take control of your own mind. You can guide it anywhere to achieve anything you want.

You have absolute power over your thoughts!

Anyone can develop the ability to control their mind. And as a reward, they gain health, inner peace, the ability to make decisions, freedom from fear and anxiety, and a positive attitude, as well as a certain quality of life and financial security.

You must know what you want and be aware of the impact procrastination has on your life. Let's see what steps you should take to get rid of it:

a) The first and most important step is to admit being a procrastinator and decide to break the habit. Make it your new goal.

b) Step number two is to have at least on actual goal (apart from breaking procrastination). Something you crave, something you long for.

c) Develop a strategy and action plan to achieve your goal. Build a list of the tasks you can start without procrastinating on them. Small, easy steps.

d) Carry out your plan. No excuses, no procrastination.

Change your daily routines that trigger procrastination. Charles Duhigg, the author of the book *The Power of Habit*, stated that each of our habits starts with a cue, some pre-action that generates the performance of the habit. For example, high tension (the cue) can lead you to overeat (the habit). Or putting on your workout clothes (the cue) triggers you to go work out (the habit). Habits are learned in earlier life. They are not innate, thus they are changeable. Duhhig talks about a third element, closing the habit creation loop — reward. Every time you do something to change your bad habits, reward yourself. But we'll talk more about this later.

The habit of procrastination started as a defense mechanism. We wanted to push the boundaries of childhood further and wanted to live carefree lives, and so we learned to procrastinate (subconsciously) as we were growing up. Procrastination was born from defiance, but turned into a habit. We developed all those bad habits that hold us in place in our comfort zones and are resistant to change. They destroy the smallest notion of change.

Take action to change these habits. Develop the habit of fighting bad habits. That's what you are doing right now. Building the habit of doing everything at the right time is a serious challenge.

If I've learned anything about self-improvement, it is that only reading about it won't get me anywhere. Only taking the time to sit down and put my thoughts in written form will make the real change. Therefore, this is the best tip I can give to you too. Sit down, take a paper and pencil, and write the following:

- Write the main goal you'd like to achieve in your life on the first page. Determine the circumstance, situation, or action that will define your idea of success when the goal is met.

- On the other side, write down and clearly define what you offer to life in exchange for achieving your goals. Write down where you plan to start giving in exchange for getting. Something for something. You don't have to think about anything unachievable here. Simple things like *"today, I'll make two people happy"* or *"today, I will help someone in need"* are more than enough.

- On a new sheet of paper, write down 5-10 tasks you will do today. This list should be a mixture of small tasks like washing the dishes and big tasks like writing a chapter of your book. You will have 5-10 new tasks to complete every day. Do not postpone small tasks and push them to the next day. For example, don't postpone taking out the trash or paying the phone bill.

1.) Pick a major task for the day, the one that you have been postponing the longest or is the most pressing.

2.) Think about the reasons you need to complete the selected task.

3.) Think about the excuses you've used for not starting it.

4.) Compare the lists from points 2 and 3. What do you think when you see the pressing reasons for completion and the excuses for delaying next to each other?

5.) Start working on the selected task. If necessary, break the process down into smaller parts. If we're talking about a task that can't be completed overnight, start with the first part of it as a daily task. If you want to write a book, for example, start with writing one chapter a day. Or one page. Start small, get into the flow of the habit, and increase the workload gradually.

6.) Once you've finished the first task, start with the second task. Don't put it off. Do not postpone it unless you literally ran out of time or energy because you underestimated the length of the previous task.

You can always be creative and develop new mechanisms to make your tasks easier. This is why we have dishwashers and cars. They are all a result of seeking long-term comfort. For example, you can pay most of your bills online these days. Take the time to open an online bank account, and learn how to pay your phone bill online instead of going to T-Mobile to pay in person every month.

"Act as if it were impossible to fail." I found this quote by Dorothea Brande in an old notebook of mine, framed in red.

Nothing is mandatory. It is up to you. You made the decision that will take you out of your comfort zone. The most effective antidote for procrastination is executing an activity that requires discipline.

What is discipline, in this context? Discipline means doing something even when you don't want to. Here is your weapon to destroy unnecessary procrastination. The first step is to:

a)   Have a to-do list.

Write down absolutely everything you need to do the next day, then prioritize the items by marking the most pressing ones URGENT. Most people who only do the urgent things during the day still become dead tired by evening.

Write down your to-do list for the next week, month, or even year, creating not just urgent but important groups. It is almost an endemic that when something is not urgent, people keep postponing it. When you get to a point that something becomes urgent, you can no longer procrastinate, but by then you've created a stressful and unhealthy environment. Concentrate on the important groups, and do every important task at the proper time to save yourself the stress of "urgency."

b) Write a not to do list.

Write down anything you don't want to do or that does not need to be done. For example:

Do not waste your time in front of the television watching shows that are not useful or that you cannot learn from. You do not need to meet people who waste your time with their meaningless conversations.

c) Divide the larger tasks into smaller parts.

To the classic question, "How do you eat an elephant?" there is the classic answer: "One bite at a time." For example, how do you write a book? You start thinking and divide the whole thing into smaller steps. Like this:

- **Task 1** — Figure out what you want to write about. Select a topic.
- **Task 2** — Summarize the book in one sentence.
- **Task 3** — Start collecting material on the chosen topic. Explore how other people feel about the matter. Read books, watch videos, listen to podcasts, talk to strangers, and take notes.

- **Task 4** — Start outlining and writing the book.
- **Task 5** — Publish the material in printed form and/or audiobook.
- **Task 6** — Promote your product.

It is good to break the work into smaller parts, because when one part is finished, you can finally cry out, "Yeah, it's done!" and feel a little success before moving on to the next step. It is a liberating feeling. The tasks that take more than an hour can be quite energy consuming. Their completion can take weeks, months, or a longer time. If this is the case, divide them into sub-tasks until they become manageable.

d) The technique of building positive statements comes from powerful questions.

What does a good and powerful question look like? Why do we care about the answer? Now that's an excellent and powerful question. Ask yourself tough, positive questions to get your brain to work on the answers. Your subconscious is the most effective partner assisting you in the battle against procrastination.

Why is ice cold? Why is the night dark? Why is the grass green? These are the questions of a small child. We grew up asking. By asking, we broadened our knowledge, our experience, and our emotions.

e)   Start with what you don't like to do, but needs to be done.

It is better to "eat the frog" and be done with the unpleasant tasks first. It's a relief, and makes the rest seem easy.

f)   Reward yourself.

Every time you check something off your to-do list — a task completed or a section finished — reward yourself. Cue — behavior — reward — these are all essential steps in building good habits. Do something that feels good and makes you happy. Keep it proportional — small task, small reward; big task, big reward.

How to Find Your Most Important Goals

The best way to uncover your most important goals is to get a piece of paper and write down the goals you have been dreaming of since you were a child. Write a maximum of ten goals. People usually have two reasons they don't actually want to write down what they want.

1. They are afraid if they write it down that someone — usually themselves — will make them accountable for it.
2. In reality, they have no concrete plans or life goals.

Write down your most important goals. Rank them in order of importance. When you have all of them, follow the instructions below.

Ask three questions about each goal. The first question's answer is the goal itself. The other two questions are auxiliary questions to broaden your perspective about the importance of that particular goal. Rank the auxiliary questions from 1-10 based on their importance. (10 is very important, one is totally meaningless.)

1. Rank the goal on a scale from one to 10. The first place is worth 10 points, second place is worth nine points and so on, down to the last place with only one point in

value. You can't give the same number twice as an answer to the question, "What is your main goal?"

2. How fulfilled would you feel if you achieved this goal? (1-10)

3. How badly would it impact you if you didn't reach this goal? (1-10)

This sounds a bit complicated, so let me illustrate the process with my own top five goals at the moment. (I will rank the goals as 10 — nine — eight — seven — six even though I have only five. Why? You'll see later.)

- Participating in a CrossFit Competition.
- Writing 50 books.
- Getting to know my mother better.

- Getting to the next level in my relationship.
- Living for three months in New Zealand.

These are my top five goals I want to reach within a given timeframe. Let's say in 2018. Now let's take them one by one:

a.) Participating in a CrossFit competition.

1. Ranking of importance: Seven.
2. How fulfilled would you feel if you achieved this goal? Seven, because CrossFit is my greatest outlet to challenge my body. Succeeding in a competition would make me feel proud of my physical capacity and resilience.
3. How badly would it impact you if you didn't reach this goal? Four, because even if I don't go to a competition, the work I put in at the gym day by day wouldn't be worthless. The fact that I didn't make it to

a competition would bother me minimally, and I can try it again and again.

b.) Writing 50 books.

1.) Ranking of importance: Eight.

2.) How fulfilled would you feel if you achieved this goal? Eight, because it would mean I really challenged my creativity and mental abilities. Furthermore, writing books is my job and passion.

3.) How badly would it impact you if you didn't reach this goal? Eight, for the same reasons — in negative — this goal would make me feel fulfilled if I succeeded.

c.) Getting to know my mother better.

1.) Ranking of importance: Nine.

2.) How fulfilled would you feel if you achieved this goal? 10, because for 25 years, my mother was almost a stranger to me. She fell ill when I was very young, and through the years, I couldn't really detach from my messed-up childhood. I saw myself as the victim, and her the reason behind my misery. Now I can be objective about her, forgive her — and myself — and try my best to create a mother-daughter relationship.

3.) How badly would it impact you if you didn't reach this goal? Nine, because time is running out. She will be 60 this year, and I am hardly ever at home. Still, I know one can't rush emotions and acceptance, so if we just made a little progress, I would be happy.

d.) Getting to the next level in my relationship.

1.) Ranking of importance: 10.

2.) How fulfilled would you feel if you achieved this goal? 10. I know, very cheesy, but I am at that age when girls really want the next step to happen, especially after almost three years of dating. Objectively, I know that a ring and eventually a paper doesn't change anything. I also know this goal doesn't entirely depend on me, but if I'm honest with myself — and I am — this might be my biggest wish at the moment.

3.) How badly would it impact you if you didn't reach this goal? Five, because I'm not in a huge rush. Considering that the time frame is 2018, I wouldn't hit absolute rock bottom if the "deadline" wouldn't be met.

- e.) Living for three months in New Zealand.
1.) Ranking of importance: Six.
2.) How fulfilled would you feel if you achieved this goal? Five, because during

my travels, I learned that it's not the place that matters, necessarily, but the people in it. New Zealand is the most beautiful country I've ever visited, so it definitely charged me with its raw, natural beauty. I'd be happy even if I lived in a cottage for three months, writing and living simply.

3.) How badly would it impact you if you didn't reach this goal? Three. Since this is a big world and I have many goals lined up before this one, and I still have the time in the world (hopefully) to go to live in New Zealand for three months, I wouldn't be too sad.

You can add more auxiliary questions to refine your quantifiable rankings. Using only the first three parameters often brings about a tie among your goals' importance. The fourth parameter could be "How urgent is this?" if you don't have a specific deadline for the goal. Find parameters that bring relevant results. If there is a tie, you can add one more criteria that can help you resolve it.

How do you rate your own survey? Divide all your important listed goals into three groups:

1. Very important — the average of all the parameters should be eight or greater (8<X)*

2. Important — the average of all the parameters should be between six and eight (6<X<8)

3. Can wait (important, but not urgent) — the average of all the parameters is less than six (X<6)

*X is the average value of the result.

How to do the math:

1) Working with three parameters

   a=10 b=9 c=9

   X=a+b+c=10+9+9=28/3=9.33

   Thus, X=9.33

   8<X=9.33

   So this is a very important goal.

Let's see the ranking of my five goals:

- Participating in a CrossFit Competition: 7+7+4= 18/3 = 6 — Important
- Writing 50 books: 8+8+8= 24/3 = 8 — Very important
- Getting to know my mother better: 9+10+9= 28/3 = 9.3 — Very important
- Getting to the next level in my relationship: 10+10+5= 25/3 = 8.3 — Very important
- Living for three months in New Zealand: 6+5+3= 14/3 = 4.6 — Can wait

As you can see, based on my calculations, there is a little change of order in the de facto importance of my goals, compared to how I ranked them initially. If I only answered just one question, namely the ranking of importance, the order would be this: relationship — mother — books — CrossFit — New Zealand. But using and ranking auxiliary questions, it turns out, fixing the relationship with my mother is the most important priority I have at the moment. If I had more auxiliary questions, my real ranking of importance would have become even more accurate.

As you can see, thinking slowly about your goals can lead you to more real and accurate answers than to listen to your snap judgment.

2. Working with five parameters for greater accuracy or because we have a tie between two

particular goals after using the first three parameters.

a=10 b=9 c=9 d=5 e=4

X=a+b+c+d+e=10+9+9+5+4=37/5=7.4

Thus, X=7.4 and 6<7.4<8 makes this goal "only" important.

Chapter 2: Productivity

The Oxford Dictionary defines productivity this way: noun. *The rate at which a worker, a company or a country produces goods, and the amount produced, compared with how much time, work and money is needed to produce them.*

How would you define productivity?

You hear this word so often when people say things like: *"I should be more productive"* or *"You should increase your productivity."* What do you think when you hear remarks like these? That you should be quicker with your work? That you should produce more in the same amount of time? That you should generate more money for the company or yourself?

Whatever it means to you, one thing is certain —
the more productive you are, whatever your
reasons, the better. So how do you maximize your
productivity? I'll tell you in this chapter.

It's About Time

You may wonder how some people always finish
their work on time, even when they have a
heavier workload than others. I'm sure each and
every one of us has a friend, co-worker, or
acquaintance who is always on time and delivers
high-quality work. If you don't know somebody
like this, then you're probably this person.

All efficient people have one thing in common: a
superpower called *mastering the use of their time*.
Everyone has 24 hours at their disposal. Some
actually use most of these 24 efficiently.

And yes, sleeping is an efficient way to use your time too. Without the right amount of sleep, it is impossible to maintain focus for long. You'd be in Zombieland all day if it weren't for Nescafe, Red Bull, and other caffeine distributors whose profit margins grow as a result of your struggle to get "into the zone." So by not sleeping enough, you increase someone's macroeconomic productivity — but not yours.

The Benefits of a Highly Unmotivated State

There are times when you are highly unmotivated to do anything. You're not in the mood to do anything. I often fall prey to a wave of disinterest like when Bruno Mars sings, "Today, I don't feel like doing anything," in *The Lazy Song*. It is completely normal to feel unmotivated. You can't burn with the brightest flame all the time.

Eventually, you'll feel like you don't want to do anything, and there's nothing wrong with that.

But there is always something to do. Even when you're unmotivated, there are "must-do" activities. Just as we saw in the chapter on procrastination, there are lots of boring tasks we put off because they are tiresome, and it does not help our sense of productivity. We can still do stuff like going to the post office, paying bills, going grocery shopping, answering emails, etc.

You may say you are not interested or thrilled about anything. Well, *that's the perfect time to do the boring things.* When you are not excited about anything else, you won't feel you are wasting your precious "in the zone" time on unproductive and dull tasks.

And as counterintuitive as it may sound, doing unproductive things in an unproductive mood actually increases your productivity. When you overcome your boredom, you're able to focus 100% on the things that move you forward without being distracted with the "must-do tasks."

If you make the effort to tackle these boring tasks instead of doing nothing during your unmotivated time, you'll realize you are actually doing something. You're not on an award-winning mission, but something is better than nothing. And this will give you a sense of satisfaction, the feeling of a day well-spent, and the kick you need to be in a more creative, motivated, and productive mood later.

The Benefits of Getting Disconnected

In the digital world, productivity is exposed to more distractions than ever. We have the Internet with its infinite rabbit hole of information, social media, and games.

how to avoid distractions
...vers, founder of CD Baby and
...author of *Anything You Want*. He states that the
best and most productive time of his life was
when he totally disconnected. Mr. Sivers
experienced the power of disconnection when he
was 22 years old and spent five months alone in a
house in Oregon. In his book, he writes: "In those
five months, I wrote and recorded over 50 songs,
made huge improvements in my instrumental
skills, read 20 books (some of which changed my
life), lost 20 pounds, and got into the best physical
shape of my life."

His next solitary adventure resulted in the
creation of CD Baby, which became a 22 million-
dollar company.

Mr. Sivers claims the reason he enjoys solitude
isn't because he dislikes people; on the contrary,
he says his best ideas come from his mind when it
is in a state of flow, when he unleashes his

creativity and excludes all the noises, news, emails, pings, and meetings.

His ultimate advice for people seeking success is to disconnect. He writes that, "Even if just for a few hours. Unplug. Turn off your phone and Wi-Fi. Focus. Write. Practice. Create. That's what's rare and valuable these days."

You may think that you don't have the time to disconnect. Tony Robbins says, "If you don't have ten minutes for yourself, you don't have a life." Yes, sometimes even 10, 20 minutes of disconnection can make a significant difference. Turn on your internal focus, listen to your thoughts, and find out why you have those specific thoughts in that moment.

Live a little bit of "you" time, then go back to work. If you can afford a few hours a day or week, let's say after work or in the weekend, even better. If you are bold or free enough, give disconnection a try for a week or a month. Even four days can make a huge difference. In the next pages, I will tell you why and how.

Be in the Moment

A few years ago, I felt overwhelmed with work. In the last one and a half years, I've written books constantly, without rest. I've read more than sixty books, I have coached people, done my own book marketing, designs, everything. So I went for a five-week holiday. I would like to emphasize the word "holiday." I travel almost all the time, but it is never a holiday. I work, and coach just the same way, only I ask for my coffee in a different language. This was a holiday. Still, my first, most memorable break lasted only four days. In mid-August 2016, I felt like I needed a rest — just a short one.

So I quickly booked a log cabin in the Romanian mountains for four days. It was located in a national reserve in an isolated village of 343 people. All I wanted was silence, peace, and no Internet. I wanted to meditate, sleep, and do nothing exciting or busy, no people, no nothing. You can imagine what it was like.

I'll never forget that trip. It opened my eyes to the fact that what you want is not always what you need. Initially, I went there to chill and be alone, but instead I met a man (the owner) who was an ex-pop star in Romania and wanted to live a more peaceful life. He spends six months every summer in Romania, in that little village of 343 people, and tries to help the community. In the winter, he teaches people to surf in Uruguay. What a life, I thought.

I wanted peace, but I needed noise. I needed that inspiring person in my life to remind me that there's nothing on that mountaintop I'm trying to reach with my relentless work. He was there, he saw it, he felt alone, and now he just longs for the journey on that mountain, and to help other climbers with directions. He impressed me. I think he is truly free, but then, who knows?

Freedom is a totally subjective state of mind. Maybe his life of freedom would be a prison of unpredictability for someone else. I went there to be alone and reflect on my life, to be in the moment, to eat simple food, enjoy the sunshine and listen to the bugs. I wanted to be free — free from my mind and my troubles.

I felt then that I wasn't capturing anything at the moment, but actually, I did. I didn't realize it at that time, but today, I feel everything that my senses could embrace back then, and it feels wonderful. And I got an excited rush too. Have you ever feared something, and then the next moment, found you loved that fear because it excited you, and it changed your opinion about yourself completely? This was paragliding for me.

While discovering the mountains, I saw some people paragliding, and there, in that moment, after thinking for only five minutes, I decided I wanted to do it. A blink. There were many first times: the first time I didn't have to consider the price; the first time I didn't hesitate and analyze every detail; the first time I didn't listen to the voice of fear in my head. I was there, in the moment. Now I realize I was 100% aware that if something went wrong up there, I'd die, and I was totally okay with it. If I could choose how to die, it would probably be by falling out of the sky toward a beautiful landscape below. It was true freedom; when I ran downhill with the expert, my legs didn't shake. I just felt now, now, *now* was the moment, and in the next one, I was in the sky, my legs and arms totally free. I screamed, I screamed as loud as I could, and it was so liberating!

All that journey, I was in the moment, but I didn't realize I was in the moment until later. Maybe people are in the moment more often than they realize. Maybe by focusing so much on the moment, we actually take away from the moment. I feel so much now. And I felt so little then. Maybe the power of memorable happiness is stronger than momentary happiness.

One thing is clear: since that journey, I got back my spirit, my desire to work, to create, to help. Not myself, initially, but others. That trip inspired me to start travelling. If I only work, I can do it anywhere in the world, I thought. But at least I meet new people, I get new stimuli, I can understand how this awesome, damned world works. I don't regret living on the road — almost one and a half years now — even though sometimes it has its dark sides. I can't see my family, I fell out of connection with my friends, I've experienced jetlag, had to get to understand a new city, discover the best location to live, and was even bitten by a monkey (no kidding). All in all, it is still a wonderful state of living, and I'm eternally grateful for it.

The productivity lessons I harvested from the cottage visit and my travels are:

-   An occasional change of scenery can help you escape the inevitable boredom of (even useful) daily routines.
-   What you want and expect is not always what you need.
-   "Life is like a box of chocolates; you never know what you're gonna get." (Forrest Gump) So be open to the possibilities and say yes to unexpected, but exciting things.
-   If you focus too intently on being in the moment, you might lose it. Being in the moment is not about consciously knowing *yes, I'm in the moment,* but about enjoying everything around us. It's best if you're not

aware that you're in the moment. It means you are actively in it and not just thinking about it.

- Every person we meet can teach us something. By meeting new people, we get perspectives on how others live and can evaluate whether we're lucky with our lives and get a boost to do things wholeheartedly, or whether we should find better options for ourselves.

- A counterintuitive lesson: skipping a few days of focusing on productivity will enhance your long-term productivity.

Optimize Your Work

Regardless of whether you're self-employed or a 9-5 worker, you need consistency. This consistency should reflect in your daily habits. Good productivity habits are predictable.

In other words, to minimize your lost time, you need to know exactly what you want to do, when do you want to do it, and approximately how much time will it take. This is one way people make the most of their time. They minimize time wasted between tasks.

You may think 15 minutes is not much time, but if you waste this amount of time eight times a day, that's two hours. If you sleep eight hours a night, it means you have 16 active hours. Two hours is too much time to be wasted thinking about what to do next. Imagine how many things you can do in two hours. If you have a clear schedule for each day (including weekends), you instantly gain 14 hours a week, which is almost another full day's active time.

Having a clear schedule is helpful for developing a routine. I have a very clear schedule, and it helps my life enormously. I have a big picture of what I want to do in the next year (how many books I want to write, how many books I want to read, which books, how many hours I can coach, etc.). I also have a monthly plan. Every Sunday, I place a Post-It note on each day of the next week with four tasks for each day. These are work-related tasks only; they do not include chores like cooking and washing the dishes.

But since I mentioned it, work optimization includes minimizing the time wasted on other, non-work-related routines — like household tasks and other obligations. First, decide how much time you are willing to sacrifice for these tasks, then stick to it. But don't forget the "something for something" rule. For example, if you don't want to spend time cooking, you can order food or eat out. The benefit is that you save the cooking and dishwashing time. Usually, it is more expensive to eat out, and if the place you choose to eat is busy, you may save only a couple of minutes.

If you don't mind cooking, but you hate going grocery shopping, there's a solution for you. There are many fresh food home delivery services that mail you all the ingredients and recipes for three to five meals for two to four people a week. It doesn't sound cheep, but the price per meal per person is usually not more than $8-$10. Because all the ingredients are fresh and more special than rice and chicken, I'd say it's a good deal. You can prepare most meals in about 40 minutes, and they are delicious.

You can optimize your work by defining your workplace. If you work in an office, it's easier, but even if you work at home or are a "digital nomad," you should be able to establish a place to work. Don't make it anything fancy. What I say is exactly what I mean: a place where you work and do nothing else. There should be no TV or other distractions. Make sure this place is comfortable, quiet, and has enough lights and clean air.

If you know that your greatest distraction is the online world, fight back with online tools to help with self-control and productivity. Follow this link http://99u.com/articles/6969/10-online-tools-for-better-attention-focus and you can read Jocelyn K. Glei's article about the 10 online tools that can help you overcome your distraction problem.

Also I recommend the products I personally use to make my yearly, monthly, and weekly schedules (apart from the Post-Its that I keep on my laptop). I bumped into Shannon F.'s work by chance on Etsy during a procrastination period when I was digging deeper and deeper into an online shopping rabbit hole. Her shop's name is *Printable Pineapple* and it has some awesome handmade calendars, planners, and even a special budget planner for the holidays. I become more organized after using these products. Find out more about them at https://www.etsy.com/shop/PrintablePineapple.

Small Tricks To Set You on Track

Oh, those mornings... when you'd only like to sleep 10 more minutes. Yes, I agree, there are few more demoralizing things than waking up early on demand. There's a big difference between this and when you don't *have* to wake up early, but you choose to. Waking up early by choice fills your heart with self-appreciation, pride, and sense of accomplishment. You are awake, it's early, and you have so many chances to make the most of your day!

Why is it so horrible to wake up when you have to go to work, then? Who knows? Maybe the fact that it is compulsory, that you do it because you're afraid of getting fired or scolded by your boss. Or maybe you do it simply because you hate doing what you have to right after you wake up.

However, there are some things you can't help — you have to do them — so instead of complaining, let's explore some solutions that can help make your mornings more endurable.

1. Put your alarm as far from your bed as possible. This is how I make sure to never wake up late or fall back to sleep. If your alarm is out of reach, you'll have to get up, walk to wherever you left it, and make it *shut up*. Finally! Phew. *That was loud*, you think. You blink twice, and slowly but surely, your engines start working.

2. Eat a quick breakfast. There are so many nutritional theories — how much you should eat, when you should eat, etc. And almost all of them contradict each other. So I'll share with you what I do, because this is the experience I trust enough to

dispense: I love to eat more in the morning, but not too much. Years ago, I read an article about eating more protein in the morning, and I tried it. It proved to be true, so I'm recommending it to you. It certainly works for me and for many other people, but we don't all function the same way, so don't take my advice for granted. Consider trying it, and if you find it beneficial, stick with it.

I usually eat the following things in the morning: a protein shake (I shake it with an Americano coffee so I can also get my caffeine dose), a protein bar (20g protein, preferably low-carb), scrambled eggs with only two yolks out of the three eggs, or oats mixed with cottage cheese and some cinnamon and honey for flavor. All these foods keep me full until lunchtime, and all of them are kickass energy boosters.

3. Try to tailor-make your work time. We are different, not only in our breakfast needs, but also regarding when we are the most productive. More and more workplaces are starting to recognize this, and some are really putting the emphasis on quality of work instead of the quantity of hours their employees spend in the office. Some offices are open to negotiating special work schedules. You never know until you ask.

   Go to your manager, boss, or whoever you report to. Some companies can't afford a raise in salaries, but if you are a good worker, instead of a raise they might be inclined to change your 9-5 shift to 10-6, 11-7 or 7-3.

4. Create your ideal work environment. This can include decorations, adding or

reducing light, increasing or decreasing the number of colleagues around you, and so on. You want to be as focused as possible; you want to make the most of your knowledge. Learn to ask for what you need. If your requests are reasonable and your company is growth-oriented, I'm sure they'll take some measures to assure the best possible environment for their workforce.

Don't be afraid or ashamed to say no. If you are in the middle of a project, a thought, or simply your relaxation time, tell your colleagues, kindly but firmly, that you need some alone time. It's not easy, at first. You may fear they'll get upset with you, but if you respect their privacy and you are normally friendly and approachable, people will respect you even more for your strong sense of self-respect.

5. Don't forget to exercise. I know, it sounds awful, especially if you cast your vote against it a long time ago. Whether you like it or not, doing physical activity is part of a healthy daily routine. Don't do something you absolutely hate, but don't put your hand on your heart and swear to yourself that you're not interested in anything.

    Is there something that if you had time, money, energy, etc., you'd gladly try? Identify what type of sport it is: competitive, team, high-intensity, low-intensity, monotonic, changeable, or something you can do at home. If you really don't have the chance to do something you'd like, try to find something similar but affordable in time, energy, and money. Be creative — today YouTube is a talking encyclopedia, and eBay is the fairy godmother who can make your wish come true quite cheaply. I'm sure you can figure out how, what, and when to work out.

6. Improve your sleeping habits. The first thing I was willing to pay money for was bed-related stuff. I have weird expectations for where I sleep — like the pillow must be memory foam, not too soft, not too hard; no polyester quilts; and if I drop a quarter on my sheet, it should bounce. Also, I need quiet and darkness. It's crazy, yes, but I know I can have a restful night's sleep if all these conditions are met. And, at least when I am at home, I like to have them.

If you feel that anything on your bed distracts you from sleep because it's uncomfortable — change it. It's a good investment. Learn what physical conditions you must have to get a good night's sleep and create them. Sometimes these changes can have a placebo effect too, like when you buy a new dress and wear it for the first time and feel much prettier in that dress than you did in your old one.

If your sleeping problems are not physical, but related to mental issues, depending on the problem you can try to change your daily routines, or in severe cases, go to a doctor or ask for professional advice. Caffeine, eating, or sitting in intense light until bedtime can, for example, increase the chance of insomnia or shallow sleeping. Also, if you eat a big meal before bed, your brain will stay active while digesting, so sleeping can be challenging.

Dr. Nitun Verma, the medical director of the Washington Township Center for Sleep Disorders in Freemont, California, has some solutions. She says we have to give our brain the "farming environment," meaning we have to stay in the dark during the night and light during the day.[i] He advises people to start dimming lights a few hours before we plan to sleep. There are some excellent lights on the market with adjustable intensity that can be a good long-term investment. It's interesting that darkness and light affects blind people's sleep too. Dr. Verma says that even if they can't see, light still stimulates nerves in the eyeball.

A last piece of sleep-related advice: Have a go-to-sleep as well as a wake-up alarm. It is more difficult to respect the bedtime than the wake-up alarm, but strengthen your resolve and include this small change in your daily routine. If you know that you'll still waste time with this and that, set a warning alarm 30 minutes before the actual bedtime alarm and another one five minutes before. After the second alarm, put down whatever you are doing, brush your teeth, and go to bed.

7. Get out in nature. We are part of nature, but in the rush of daily life, we tend to overlook this important fact. Research has proven that walking in a forest or on a shore, taking a nap in a hammock in a park, or simply enjoying the birds' singing can significantly reduce stress and improve creative thinking and memory. A study

conducted by the Dutch National Survey of General Practice concluded that people who live in a 1-3km (0.6-1.8 miles) radius of a green area had less stress and perceived or actual health problems.

Another study conducted by Robert Ulrich at Texas A&M University proves that adding flowers or green plants to your office increases creativity significantly. This study lasted for eight months and resulted in a 15% increase in ideas from male workers, and more flexible, problem-solving skills with female employees.[ii] For more interesting researches, facts, and curious stories, visit http://www.bakadesuyo.com.

Tips From The Tip of the Mountain

Everybody does it differently. As long as you make some changes to improve your daily routines and build better habits, it doesn't matter which tips from this book you choose to implement. I try to show you as many options as possible so you can choose the ones that are the most fitting, helpful, or relevant to your day. You are seven billion; I am one. It is very hard to find solutions that can work for everyone, so I've decided to give many options from different perspectives to give you a greater chance of finding something valuable and applicable.

I read a lot. Often, I read a great book that goes into depth on one topic or solution. Most of the time, I find these in-depth explanations to be interesting and thoughtful, but I can hardly ever apply them to my life. However, when I read a book that has a main topic and presents a variety of solutions, I can pick which ones I know will fit my life and then search out a more in-depth book on that particular topic.

So, in the following pages, I'll present you with some tactics that world-famous people use to make their daily routines better.

1. Jack Dorsey

    The CEO of Square and co-founder of Twitter is a busy guy. He has two huge companies to oversee, and decided to work eight hours a day, Monday to Friday, on each one. Yes, that's 16 hours a day, five days a week. When I grow up, I don't think I want to be Jack Dorsey.

    Before we start fundraising and donating our free hours to Mr. Dorsey, I'd like to add that he worked these intense hours for only a limited time, and right now he is more focused on Square. But how did he manage to keep it together when he was working 16-hour days?

He themed his days. He developed a strict structure of daily and weekly routines for both his companies and followed this structure with steadfast discipline. Every weekday, he spent time on one particular area or aspect of his businesses. On Mondays, he worked on management, on Tuesdays, he focused on products, and so on.

If you feel your schedule is tight, especially if you're an entrepreneur, you could try this system. It gives you a structured and predictable weekly routine and lifts the weight of decision fatigue from your shoulders. There will always be distractions and interruptions in your daily theme, but be prepared and don't lose track of the essential task of the day, and when the distraction goes away, be ready to continue where you left off.

2. Tim Ferriss

We could say that Tim Ferriss, author of *The 4-Hour Workweek,* is the opposite of the Jack Dorsey and his 16-hour workdays. If you read his book, you'll know that Mr. Ferriss' life wasn't always as easy as a four-hour workweek would sound — quite the contrary. But with resourcefulness and a lot of hard work, he developed systems for himself that allowed him to have more free time and a relaxed lifestyle.

So what advice does he have on daily routines and habits? Nothing. Why? Because he doesn't have one. His routine is to not have a routine, and to keep everything flexible. His daily routine is

105

never the same — he does what he wants on any particular day. He has, however, some ground rules, like no phone calls or appointments on Fridays and Mondays, so he can have long weekends whenever he wants. He doesn't have extravagant programs and systems, but he does cherish his freedom of choice, and so he does most of his work in minimal time, thereby maximizing his output.

3. Evan Williams

Just for the sake of finding middle ground between Jack Dorsey and Tim Ferriss, I present the daily routine of Evan Williams, co-founder of Twitter, Blogger, and Medium.

He leaves his office midday every day to visit the gym. I mentioned previously that we are not the same when it comes to productivity or most active hours. Mr. Williams realized it's not very productive for him to be at the gym in the morning. He found he is more productive at work in the morning, but loses focus in the middle of the day. So he decided to go to the office early and take a two-hour midday break to go to the gym. He gets refreshed at the gym and also breaks the monotony so when he returns to the office, he can concentrate with a fresh mind again.

If you can swing it, try taking a midday break to do something totally different — train, exercise, or do something else that gives you pleasure. Return to working one or two hours later and you'll feel the difference.

Chapter 3: Philosophy

When we think about changing daily routines and habits, we usually think about certain actions, but all our actions are the result of our thoughts. These thoughts elicit feelings and emotions, and based on these emotions, we take actions. This is called the TEA model: thoughts, emotions, and actions. All of us function based on these three human manifestations. I'd like to add a fourth element; this element is the result of the previous three.

Does this make TEA model the TEAR model? Let's hope they are tears of joy, not sadness. All jokes aside, if we want to understand what is currently happening in our lives and where our results come from, the equation would be: thoughts + emotions + actions.

Thus, the key to changing your daily routines and habits permanently is not found in how many times you repeat something, or in how positively or negatively you feel for them, but in what you think about them. In order to make the changes in your daily routine last, you have to change your thoughts.

According to neuro-linguistic programming (NLP), the thoughts that elicit our emotions are "sponsoring thoughts" in opposition to conscious thoughts that make up the context of the way we perceive the world. [iii] Everything else in our internal landscape, our conscious thoughts, our emotions, our beliefs, come from profound contexts that we viewing the world through. If we change the context, not only will the thoughts change, but so will the emotions and abilities we have inside us.

It is important to have a philosophy for living your life. Some people don't; they just fly around following the current "trends." Without a philosophy, it is difficult to determine life goals. Without goals, it is almost impossible to build routines that lead you to your goals — because you don't have any, right? Or even if you have a vague inclination toward something you consider a goal, if it is not rooted in a deep belief, it won't last long, and neither will the related routines.

What do you believe in? What is your philosophy on life? What do you base your life decisions on? What habits do you wish to acquire? Why? How important is that habit for you? What goal can that habit help you accomplish?

If you look at the other side of the coin, you could say that if you lack life goals, you also lack a clear philosophy in life. That's right, it works the other way around as well. If you don't believe in anything, if you don't have certain expectations from life, and you don't have any values that you cherish, you'll float on the wind like an empty plastic bag. When you are on your deathbed, you will look back and realize that you wasted your chance to make your life count. You didn't go for something that would have been valuable; instead, you wasted it because you let distractions dominate your life.

Whatever philosophy of life you embrace, your life will be better than if you tried to live without one. Don't think about anything complicated here. It's not like you have to read all the great works from great thinkers, or that you must adopt one philosophy 100%. Just have a clear vision of life's guidelines and the values you want to follow.

Back to our topic of daily routines and habits — if you feel you're not in a satisfactory place right now, then maybe you should consider that this could be the result of following a deficient, wrong, or nonexistent philosophy.

In the following chapter, I will present you with different philosophies and values gathered from my readings. They can all lead you to a successful life. Based on your core values, you can consider undertaking or adopting some of them.

Anti-Passion Mindset

I recently re-read Cal Newport's book *So Good They Can't Ignore You* about how to become successful in your job and how to create the life you want. His advice is almost the opposite of what we usually hear. Most of the time, we hear advice on how to follow our passion, to leave our

jobs, and to stop the grind and create ourselves.[iv]
Well, Mr. Newport thinks differently, and this doesn't mean he is wrong. Moreover, his thoughts are worth reading for everybody who has a passion-oriented life philosophy (I'm one of those people). It's always good to know the alternatives to our beliefs, as well as the thoughts that challenge our beliefs.

Regarding your career, the path to happiness is more complex than simply asking yourself:

What should I do with my life?

Following your passion is not the best advice when you think about creating the career of your dreams. According to Mr. Newport, the "follow your passion" conventional wisdom is wrong. The passion-oriented career philosophy not only fails to describe how exactly people can end up working their dream jobs, but also, for most people, it can actually make life worse by leading them to a frequent job shifting lifestyle, as well as low income and high anxiety levels.

Now, you may think that if "follow your passion" is not good advice, what should you do?

Passion has no direct impact on creating a fulfilling work life. So instead of following your passion, let it follow you in your search "to become so good that they can't ignore you."

Stop focusing on finding the right work. Instead, focus on working right, and gradually learn to love what you do. Cal Newport states that the more years you spend doing your job and the better you become at it (due to experience and diligence), the more you'll consider it a calling. The more experience, expertise, and praise you receive, the more you'll grow to love what you do. The longer you stick with something and the better you become, the more passionate you'll feel about it.

In Mr. Newport's analysis, hard work and excellence come first and may be followed by passion, but not vice versa. You might wonder how you will find the motivation to stick with what you do if you hate it. You understand that following your passion means you'd start from zero (or very little) real world experience. Still, I'd find doing that easier than grinding to the point where I'd label my current job as my passion.

His book answers this question. Scientists figured that instead of finding a way of "matching work to pre-existing ability, interests, passions, or personality," you should motivate yourself by taking the following three psychological needs into consideration:

- autonomy
- competence

- relatedness[v]

What does this mean? Autonomy is the feeling of having control over your life, competence is the aforementioned feeling that you are good enough in what you do, and relatedness stands for the satisfactory connection you have with other people. In other words, try to develop a relatively flexible work schedule (you can do it by following the advice in the previous chapter), and work in you ideal productivity time zone to help you improve the quality of your work and the ability to deeply focus on what you do. And, last but not least, avoid energy vampires and maintain good relationships with your colleagues. It can be a serious deal breaker if you hate your job because you hate the people you are supposed to cooperate with.

According to Mr. Newport, the problem with the "follow your passion" philosophy is that when people adopt it, they become convinced that there's a magical job waiting for them out there somewhere, and when they find it, their lives will instantly become meaningful. Unfortunately, in most cases, it is not a "when" but an "if." If they fail to find this job but continue to search for a life with meaning, they turn to the dark side of chronic job switching and fall into a deep pit of self-loathing.

In order to get something worthy and valuable, you have to give something worthy and valuable in exchange — this is the experience and rare expertise you develop over years of working. To be considered great at your work does not just require courage, but also skills.

But as with any rule, Mr. Newport's thesis has certain exceptions. There are times you shouldn't apply the "craftsman mindset," as he calls his alternative to passion mindset. These exceptions are in the following cases:

- when the job you do has few or no opportunities to distinguish yourself with relevant skills;
- when the job is in opposition to your core values, or you think about it as useless, or even harmful;
- you have to share your work with people you don't like and can't relate to.

I wanted to present Cal Newport's philosophy because it offers a great alternative to the conventional "follow your passion" mindset. Trying to look at your career from this perspective can be difficult in the beginning, but long-term, it can bring you happiness and satisfaction. In any case, excelling at what you already know is less stressful than chasing something that has no guarantee.

Depending on what your main value is, if having peace of mind is more important than seeking adventure, adopting Cal Newport's philosophy can help you create better daily "action" routines.

The Stoic Way of Living a Good Life

What is the core value of your life?

The stoic answer for that is whatever you hold dear, you're unlikely to have a happy and meaningful life if you don't overcome your insatiability. And when it comes to happiness, according to the stoics, you'll be the happiest when you learn to find joy in what you have and in what comes from within.

Our unhappiness is rooted in our insatiable nature. We want to become happy due to something external — let's say a promotion, or buying a new car. We start working hard to achieve this goal, but when we get it, we instantly lose interest. We want something else instead, something even bigger. This doesn't mean that we shouldn't want more, or that we shouldn't strive to become better, but it means we need to learn how to appreciate what we have, rather than continuously trying to catch the future.

The easiest and best way to achieve happiness is to want the things you already have.

In *A Guide to the Good Life: The Ancient Art of Stoic Joy*, William Irvine describes the most important values stoicism teaches us. Following Cato, Seneca, and Marcus Aurelius' work, Mr. Irvine created a great and easy-to-follow book about stoicism. For the sake of completeness, I recommend you read his book. If you are more interested in stoicism, read the aforementioned ancient geniuses' works also. There's a lot in these books when it comes to following a life-changing philosophy.[vi]

One of the core values of stoic philosophy is self-discipline. Why should you work on possessing it?

Because having control over your thoughts, and thus your actions, can help you determine what you want to do with your life. With a lack of self-discipline, you have to walk a path determined by someone else.

Tranquility is another state highly praised by the stoics. It is a psychological state in which people experience negative emotions like grief, anxiety, and fear, but also positive emotions, like joy.

According to Seneca, you have to learn to use your reasoning ability to get rid of all that intrigues or scares you. Accept that the world is bipolar — good and bad coexist. If you expect only good, your life will be stressful and sad. The more you can adopt this reasoning, the more tranquility and freedom you'll have in your life.

I can say that it is often part of our daily routines to take what we have for granted -- our jobs, our well-equipped kitchens, our bank accounts, even the air we breathe and the health we have. Stoics encourage us to change this daily routine by thinking about and practicing poverty. They encourage us to start thinking about losing everything we take for granted — our health, including our ability to speak, walk, swallow; our family; wealth; or freedom. How would you feel if you lost your ability to speak, hear, walk, breathe, and swallow? How would you feel if you lost your freedom?

This is not negative thinking, but a sure way to enhance the feelings of gratitude toward what we owe. These are the greatest values of life, and we don't even think about them, and we do very little to cherish them. Instead, we chase empty, valueless objects and objectives.

If you allow for many pleasures in your life and try to live as comfortably as possible, nothing will seem bearable when a crisis comes. This is not because that crisis is too much to bear, but because you are soft. Make sure you never get too comfortable. This way, you'll be able to appreciate comfort better and be happier when you get it.

If you expose yourself to self-chosen discomfort from time to time, you'll be more able to handle hard times that bring true discomfort. You could also say that you'll have a larger comfort zone in regard to unpredictable or bad events.

Exposing yourself to discomfort includes dealing with annoying people. When someone's behavior upsets you, reflect for a few minutes on your own shortcomings. If you do this, you will become more empathetic to others and realize that often, what you find annoying about others may be something you do also. What upsets people is not the facts themselves, but their judgments on these facts. Also, refusing to respond to an insult is one of the most effective reactions.

One of the main values of the 21st century is fame, and people often pursue it. Everybody has different reasons for wanting it, and aspirations for their desired level of fame. Some want worldwide fame, some only regional or workplace popularity, but almost everyone seeks the admiration of others. But the price of fame, more often than not, is so great that it exceeds any benefits.

So if you consider seeking fame as a core value that you want to build your daily routines, or your life, around, know that it is an infidel companion. Fame is like the consumer society: it stays only until you make your first mistake. Then it shows up somewhere else. If you seek social status, basically you're making it your goal to please others, not yourself. Rather, try to be indifferent to what people think of you — not only regarding their disapproval, but also their approval. Cato consciously did or said things to trigger the contempt of others only so he could practice ignoring their contempt.

A stoic philosophy seems to be difficult to adopt in our money-oriented world. However, if you learn to simplify your life just a little based on these ancient wisdoms, you'll become much happier. As a daily habit, introduce days of low modern stimuli.

For example, decide that every Saturday you'll disconnect from the world, and that you'll try to live as people lived before television, Internet, or telephones were invented. You can also practice poverty; have a set of very cheap and low-quality clothes and consciously wear them one day a month while you eat cheap food and only drink water. Try going into the cold underdressed, or into the rain without an umbrella or raincoat. Learn to value the things you have. And to be able to truly value them, you have to experience what it would be like to lose them.

Chapter 4: Focus

Do you ever find yourself losing focus? One night, I was at a work dinner and my mind kept wandering. I had a bunch of things I needed to get done that night, and I simply couldn't focus on what was being said by all of my coworkers. Obviously, this wasn't the best situation to put myself in. As much as I tried to focus, their voices were like the teachers from Charlie Brown. All I heard was mumbling and noise, with zero comprehension lasting in my mind.

It was so bad that one of my coworkers stopped mid-story and asked, "Are you listening?" Immediately feeling like a student being chastised by a teacher, I exclaimed, "Yes! Please, continue," before drinking a whole glass of water and nodding when I was supposed to during the tale. It was miserable. If I had just picked up on some simple things to help increase my focus, I would have been saved a load of embarrassment.

Unfortunately, this happens to a lot of us quite often. We try to focus on something at hand, but it doesn't work. Focusing is hard. With devices demanding our attention, our crazy, busy lives, and the people we are with, it can be hard to dial down and focus. Thankfully, there are some tried and true methods that can really help you to focus in the long run. And, they are backed by science. This isn't some hoax about what will and won't work; these are proven techniques which can help you change your focus by doing a few simple things.

The Power of the Chewing Gum

What if I told you that chewing gum could actually help your focus? I know, something as simple as gum doesn't seem like it could really help, but it actually can. Whether you're a bubble gum lover or a spearmint-obsessed chewer, any kind of gum can help you to improve your focus. This is actually something that has been studied in depth among researchers. If something that costs pennies could improve focus, wouldn't you want to use it?[vii]

In the *British Journal of Psychology,* researchers found that chewing gum helps focus because it increases the amount of oxygen that flows to the parts of the brain that are responsible for attention. More oxygen improves your brain's function, so it could literally save you from daydreaming during that important class or meeting you're attending.[viii]

Another study performed by Lucy Wilkinson and Andrew Scholey found that gum gives your insulin levels a small spike, which gives your brain an added energy boost and improves long-term memory. This is all just from chewing gum!

If you aren't completely convinced, don't worry. I'm not done yet. Another team of psychologists at St. Lawrence University did a study about how chewing gum would affect a group of individuals during demanding cognitive tasks. There were 159 students that were given these tasks. Things like logic puzzles, random number sequences, and other challenging brain games were required in this study. Half of the group got gum and half of the group didn't. The group that was given gum was separated further into sugar-free gum and sugar-added gum.

What researchers found was that in five out of six different tests, the group that was chewing the gum outperformed the group that wasn't.

However, whether the gum was filled with sugar or not didn't matter. You could potentially chew any type of gum you want and perform better during the day while working or attending something important. Just by grabbing your favorite flavor, you increase your focus. If you want to develop good focus habits, start out by trying to chew some gum. While you don't want to rely on it for the rest of your life, it can really help you out in a pinch. [ix]

The Sound of Silence

If you're not a huge gum chewer, there are other alternatives to making your focus better and stronger. One way to improve your focus is to engage in something we all probably know, but many of us don't like to do.

Quiet time.

Being in silence has been shown to be better for our focus. Now, I know what a lot of you are thinking. Many of us claim that it is impossible to get work done in the silence because our mind wanders too much during it. I'm not necessarily talking about some soothing music in the background. Although, that could also distract you. I'm talking about ambient noise, like cars honking their horns, kids screaming outside, and other noises that you don't necessarily expect to happen. This releases the stress hormone, cortisol, which according to the former director of Lake Erie College of Osteopathic Medicine, Mark A.W. Andrews, can hinder your ability to focus and do good work. And it gets worse the more noise you hear.[x]

If you live on a busy street in New York, horns honking are probably second nature to you. But that doesn't mean they don't still affect you. You need to design your workspace to reflect the ambient noise so it doesn't disturb your work in its entirety. Maybe this means you need to embrace the noise. Choose some relaxing music that you know you can tune out and focus through. The music can stop the sudden noises from grabbing your attention, and you can remain focused throughout it.

Or work somewhere else. Places like libraries are often very quiet, and you can even blend in with the smooth tones of a local coffee shop. Using these noises to your advantage will help you to focus better.

If you work remotely like me, you can rent a working space. There are buildings specified to offer you this facility. You pay an amount of money monthly, but in return, you get a polished office, free coffee — in better places, even Cheerios — and you can work in peace and quiet. It is also proven through research that it is healthy to separate your workspace from your home. So if you have a home office, work remotely, or have your own business without an office, renting a workspace is not only a good idea noise-wise, but also psychologically. To put it simply, it is easier to leave your work-related problems at the office if you actually have one.

The Good Old Meditation

Speaking of quiet, another way to increase your focus is with a little bit of meditation. The *Psychological Science* journal recently came out with a study that showed meditation can help people to focus their attention on whatever task it is that they are doing — even if it is incredibly boring.

It was led by Katherine MacLean of UC Davis and included twelve other researchers. They noticed that almost everyone gets tired after concentrating on a task. It exerts a lot of brain power, and the exhaustion sets in. The boring task that the participants had to do was to watch lines pop up on a computer screen. Whenever a smaller line popped up, they had to press down on their mouse. It was incredibly boring, and that was the point of it all. However, some of the participants had meditated at the retreat before this task.

Those who had meditated were much better at seeing the subtle differences in the lines, and their ability to find the smaller lines increased with the amount of meditation they were doing. This study showed that meditation can help you to focus and perform better, but there was one caveat. The meditators didn't react any faster to the tasks than those who hadn't meditated. While they were more accurate and better at it, they were not faster.[xi]

Doodling Mood

There are so many of benefits of meditation, but so many of us refuse to do it, regardless. If you fall into that boat, doodling might be a better way to help you focus. Jackie Andrade performed a study asking the participants to doodle through the recordings. The ones who doodled while listening to the recordings had a much higher retention level than those who were not doodling.[xii]

We used to get chastised for doodling in elementary school, but it actually helped us to increase our focus. Doodling takes just enough of our attention that we don't wander off into daydreams, so we stay focused on the task at hand. These can be doodling simple lines or small pictures, but it should help you focus more on what you are hearing. Obviously, there are some times when doodling won't work. When your vision is needed, you'd be better off trying out a different focus habit than doodling. However, if you're in on a phone meeting or just need to listen to something, doodling can help to make things clearer, easier to understand, and give you a better retention rate.

The Magic of Nature

When I was a kid, I lived in the countryside among green fields, rushing rivers, chickens, cows, and bugs. I felt I was one with the nature. After the age of 14, I became a big city girl, which meant that I would spend a bunch of time inside stuffy buildings. I would spend hours upon hours sitting in lectures, studying in my dorm, and then socializing indoors. Even though there was plenty to see and do outdoors, I stayed inside. It wasn't until my second semester that I realized something had to change.

It was overwhelming, being surrounded by walls all the time. It was like my own private prison, and I suddenly felt claustrophobic and not ready to spend another minute inside. I took a deep breath and decided to venture outdoors, unsure of what I would find. Thankfully, the winter was melting away and a few cherry blossom trees had started to bloom with the warm spring air. I wasn't sure what I wanted to do outdoors, but just the feeling of being outside left me refreshed. It was a bit later that I decided to take a walk around campus and then settle into one of the outdoor picnic tables to finish my studying. After that, I was hooked. Any moment I could spend outside was a good moment. I felt relieved and rejuvenated, and my work reflected it. The assignments I turned in were better, and studying became easier. The tranquil sounds of nature had gotten to me, and I felt like I had missed out on nature by not discovering it until now.

Our lives are busy; no one will say otherwise. But because of this, we don't spend a lot of time indoors. From businessmen to stay-at-home moms, we all spend too much time cooped up inside our homes and offices. The stale air creeps into our lungs, and it can be the cause for a multitude of diseases. We all know that we should spend some time outdoors to get that vitamin D from the sun, but how often do we really do it? Instead, we pop some vitamins and hope that will help us live out our lives.

It turns out that there's a pretty big reason you should be spending more time outdoors. Believe it or not, looking at green stuff is beneficial. And where can you find green stuff? Outdoors! In a study done at the University of Melbourne, Kate Lee and a group of researchers looked at how interrupting a tedious or attention-demanding task with a 40-second micro break would affect the results. The micro break they used was having the participants look at a picture of a green roof. What they found was that just looking at this green roof improved focus and performance on the task. The participants also made fewer mistakes.[xiii]

So while looking at something green can help to improve your focus, there's nothing better than looking outside and seeing some trees. However, if you can't get up and walk around to get this break to work for you, consider adding a few plants or succulents to your home or office to bring nature to you. It's a simple thing that can help you to feel more grounded and at peace.

Natural Lights

Another way to bring nature to you is to work in natural light. We are under the scrutiny of artificial light all day long, and it isn't good for us. Northwestern University did a study that found a correlation between the lighting the person used and how well they slept, their activity levels, and their quality of life. The employees who worked in natural light slept an additional 46 minutes a night, slept more soundly, and reported a higher quality of life.

Not having natural light can mess with your body's circadian rhythm. This is what tells you it is time to sleep and wake during the day and night. It's also responsible for alerting you about meal times and other daily activities. Disruptions to this can cause abnormal sleep patterns, but it can also cause depression and lethargy. It is a serious concern for many, and just switching out your lighting can help to reduce this problem.[xiv]

A study published in *The Responsible Workplace* concluded that windows were the number one deciding factor of the occupants' level of satisfaction with the building. Just imagine how much better you feel when there is a window near to you, as opposed to you sitting in a room with no windows at all. Natural lighting makes happier workers because it affects our mood and behavior. There were also fewer illnesses found in people who were exposed to natural light during the day, and that increases efficiency and productivity levels as well. Bright light can also help to reduce cortisol levels, something that is responsible for our stress.[xv]

If you have a window near you, open the blinds and let the sun shine on your workplace. However, if you aren't near a window, try and take a few breaks during the day where you can go outside and sit for a moment in the sunshine. It will help you perform better, but it will also make you a much happier person. And who is anyone to argue with that, right?

Go Green

As I mentioned briefly earlier, plants are another way to increase productivity and bring nature to you. There was a study conducted in the Netherlands and UK that randomly assigned employees to work with some plants in their vicinity. The ones who had a plant near them outperformed the employees who didn't have any access to plants. It seems silly, but there are actually a lot of reasons as to why plants can help us to feel better.

Humans used to spend a lot of time outdoors, and only recently has that changed. Plants are a way to connect with the past and still feel like we can be outside. There's more to it than that, though. Plants can also improve air quality because they literally suck some toxins from the air. This leads to a perception that the air quality is better because of plants, but it also makes the environment more visually appealing. There's nothing that a few flowers or succulents can't do to liven up a room. What goes from a boring office cubicle then turns into a wonderful oasis that is filled with fresh and clean air because of the plants around you. Plus, you don't even have to have them right next to you. Just seeing a plant is close to you can help you perform better during the day. There's no reason to say no to having plants near you![xvi]

Oh, Those Cute YouTube Videos

Last, but certainly not least, is a method that can help you perform better throughout the day. You'll never believe it... but looking at baby animals can actually improve your focus and performance. I know, you're probably thinking this is a bunch of nonsense, but I'm not joking here!

We all love baby animals, so rejoice in the fact that there are benefits from looking at them. In a Japanese research paper, *The Power of Kawaii: Viewing Cute Images Promotes a Careful Behavior and Attentional Focus,* researchers found that looking at cute images at work can help boost your attention and overall performance. Three groups of students played a game, and then looked at a few images before playing the game again. The group that had to look at baby animals outperformed their peers by a very significant margin. Apparently, it could be connected to a nurturing instinct that we all seem to have. Something about those cute animals just makes it difficult for us to *not* pay attention.[xvii]

We've all been on the Internet and have cooed over the adorable baby animals, but now you don't need to feel bad about it if you're sneaking a peek at the baby panda at work. If anyone walks in to say something, tell them that science has actually proved that looking at baby animals improves your performance. Sure, they might think you're a little nutty, but it's the truth! Between all of these different little ways to improve your performance, you should be a working machine when you need to focus on a task.

Chapter 5: Multitasking vs. Monotasking

Women are the ultimate multitaskers. If you're a woman, you know this. Going from thing to thing just seems to work... until it doesn't.

There was one day that I had a ton to do. I had a large work assignment due that night, I needed to get some laundry done, I'd promised a friend I would watch her dog, and I was dealing with trying to make dinner and look presentable for my date later that night. I knew I had to get my work assignment done before the date, but I was all over the place. I started a load of laundry, ran to my computer to type a few things while the machine filled with water, ran back to the washer to put in the detergent and start the cycle, did my makeup while listening to the notes about my work assignment, and boiled water for the pasta I was going to eat.

Turns out, things don't work that great when you try to multitask like that. There I was, doing my mascara after putting in the pasta, and I smelt something burning. Knowing that it's pretty hard to burn pasta, I blamed it on an upstairs neighbor in my apartment building. They'd probably burnt popcorn or something. I continued with my makeup and checked the time. I ran into the kitchen, knowing my pasta was going to be soggy and overcooked, but I found a much larger disaster waiting for me.

Yes, it is very hard to burn pasta, but the pasta water boils over all the time. I wasn't expecting it to in my large pot, but it did. Since some of the water got into the stove, and the burner bubbled the starchy water into a black, unidentifiable liquid. So now I was screwed. I needed to salvage my pasta to eat, scrub my stove, finish my makeup, switch the laundry to the dryer, do my work assignment, and somehow go on my date within an hour.

Multitasking was not a new experience for me, but suddenly it became my worst enemy. I vowed from that point forward that I needed to slow down and try taking each task one at a time. Multitasking is a myth. You don't stay focused on one thing, so you end up performing worse on the rest of the tasks because you were all over the map. It's not fun, and it's certainly not pretty. According to the Institute at Carnegie Mellon University, it can take up to 25 minutes just to regain your focus after becoming distracted.

With multitasking, you're distracted like no other. It's overwhelming, and you definitely cannot stay focused on the task at hand because you are trying to balance three hundred other tasks!

In a paper titled *Why is it so Hard to do My Work?* Sophie Leroy introduced a concept called "attention residue." Lots of people multitask, and it's often a fact of life in businesses. However, when you switch from one task to the other, part of your attention remains with that first task. Even if you finish the first task and quickly hop to something else, your attention remains a little. That's why it is called "attention residue." Unfortunately, studies conducted by the author showed that the more attention residue left behind with another task, the worse you perform on the future task. [xviii]

If you're spending your time switching from task to task, nothing is getting handled or done correctly. Just like with my story, I couldn't finish anything, and everything that I did was pretty bad. I mean, I burned pasta. Who else can say they've done that?

You're just spending your time and energy focusing on switching from task to task, which is a total waste. A Stanford researcher named Clifford Nass looked at the performance of multitaskers in the workplace and analyzed their ability to work well. The study participants were split into two groups. One group was a low multitasking group, and the other group was a high multitasking group. The first experiment went off without a hitch, and the researchers thought that the high multitaskers might actually be onto something. Perhaps they had better memories and could work despite their distractions because of their improved memory.[xix]

Unfortunately, the second test proved that all wrong. The deeper into the task that the high multitaskers got into, the worse they performed. The low multitaskers were doing awesome, but the ones who multitasked frequently were performing horribly. It turns out that the multitaskers can't ignore anything. While this might seem like a good thing, it is far from it. Instead of ignoring what didn't need to be seen, the multitaskers couldn't. They stored everything, which then made them perform even worse.

Basically, this means that the multitaskers cannot determine what is and what isn't needed in a task. They have a problem with relevance, and they are slowed down immensely by information that shouldn't concern them. Hungarian psychologist Mihaly Csikszentmihalyi said that refusing to multitask can get you into the best type of working, which is when you reach flow. When you're in flow, you have complete concentration on what you're working on, a clarity of goals, an understanding of time, a rewarding experience, you work effortlessly, you strike a good balance between challenge and skill, there's no self-conscious rumination, and you experience a feeling of control over the current task. [xx]

Obviously, flow is what we all desire when we are striving to work, and we get in there by focusing. You have to slash multitasking for you to acquire the focus that will bring you into flow. You know that feeling when you're just in the zone?

One day, I was so excited to write that I sat down and literally wrote dozens of pages. I didn't even know if it would turn out to be amazing, but I couldn't stop writing. It was actually pretty impressive, because I don't stay focused very well at times. The words flowed effortlessly, and I finally felt like I was getting somewhere with my writing. When I finished with that experience, I was wishing that I could summon that feeling whenever and wherever I was in life. I learned later on that this was what was considered to be flow.

When we want to work to the best of our ability, we need to focus and we need to up our performance. It can definitely be hard some days, but many of us don't even try. We go throughout our day like normal, living our lives, doing our tedious tasks, and then starting the next day in the same exact way. Can you honestly say you've tried your hardest to focus and get into that flow type work environment? Most of us just don't even think about it. We know that we need to get our stuff done, so we do what we have to do. However, it could be so much easier if we just learned how to focus and live our life so that our work wasn't hard, but effortless.

Cal Newport has a concept that is called deep work. Basically, deep work is professional activities that are preformed in a state of distraction-free concentration. They push your cognitive capabilities to their limit. This might seem overwhelming or scary, but it actually doesn't need to be tedious at all. Deep work can be creative and enjoyable — even thought-provoking or meditative. Deep work definitely gets more done with a better performance level, and incorporating it into your daily routine doesn't need to be exhausting.[xxi]

First, you can work deep work into your schedule by working deeply. Make sense? Believe it or not, it is actually pretty self-explanatory. Lots of college kids pull all-nighters to study for that exam in the morning. This is especially true around finals time, and those students are zoned in on their textbooks. You could probably tell them that some famous celebrity was outside the library handing out free donuts and they would still be reading their book. Okay, maybe not, because let's be honest — we'd all run outside for a free donut from Leonardo DiCaprio.

But working deeply is a simple equation that work accomplished = (time spent) x (intensity).

Work with a lot of intensity and stay in your zone for 90 minutes. You can slowly build this up over time to reach two to four hours, maybe even more.

Another way to incorporate this phenomenon into your life is by protecting your time. Keep a ritual or routine that is special to you that will get you prepared for going into that zone of deep work. You can schedule when you decide you're going to do deep work, or keep a tally of the hours that you spend working when or when you've reached a certain milestone. This could be finishing a client portfolio or hitting your word count for the day. Whatever it is, this is like a small motivation to show you that you are doing good work, which is deep work.

The reason this is so important is because you can get so much more done in this time period of deep work. You could spend hours doing one task while you aren't focused, or you could get in the zone and knock it out in a matter or minutes. It's simple, really, and it helps you to get more work done. Plus, it is definitely anti-multitasking. Deep work only works when you're working on one project, which is why you only need to stay in the zone for a few hours. Incorporating this into your schedule can literally help keep you sane! You'll never burn pasta again.

At least, not because you were multitasking.

Chapter 6: 50 Quick Daily Routine and Habit Changes

1. Slow down.

2. Stop once a day to admire something around you.

3. Find the positive equivalent of all your negative thoughts. (Example: Life's hard — life's easy. I can't do it — I can do it.)

4. Make walking your daily routine. Walk for at least 30 minutes each day just for the sake of walking.

5. One apple a day keeps the doctor away. Did you know that ripe apples smile? After you eat them, they transfer their smile to you.

6. Drink at least 2 liters (68 fl. Oz) a day.

7. Start your morning with a tall glass of room temperature water.

8. Learn to meditate, and do it for at least 10 minutes before sleeping.

9. Use the evening meditation to forgive yourself and others.

10. Spend time in nature. The more, the better.

11. Smile, and the world will smile back at you.

12. Have a heartfelt laugh each day.

13. Give at least three compliments a day.

14. Look in the mirror and tell yourself that you're beautiful.

15. Call your mother. (Or father, son, daughter, or anyone close to you.)

16. Read something new for 10-15 minutes each day.

17. Find the possibilities around you. See opportunities where others don't.

18. Choose to master a skill and dedicate a few minutes to it each day.

19. Search for the lesson in each failure.

20. Before making an important decision, think about two more reasons why you should or shouldn't do it, besides the obvious.

21. Focus on the solution, not the problem.

22. Stretch every morning.

23. Create your success. Don't expect it to find you.

24. Ask questions frequently.

25. Instead of judging people, try to find common ground with them.

26. If you did something wrong, apologize quickly and move on. Don't look for excuses, but don't hate yourself.

27. Don't try to be busy. That's a sign of a life that lacks organization and control.

28. Use what you have now instead of procrastinating a day with the hope that you'll be better tomorrow.

29. Step one is not the planning and preparation. Step one is hands-on action.

30. There is no "right time." There is only now or never.

31. Don't let your life stop and start. Flow.

32. Take calculated risks.

33. Be proactive instead of reactive.

34. Improve your communication skills.

35. Improve your emotion handling skills.

36. Identify your core values and act according to them.

37. Help someone else each day.

38. Don't take anything for granted.

39. Practice poverty at least one day a month — eat cheap food, wear old clothing. See your greatest fears became reality and realize they are not as horrible as they may seem.

40. The strongest and smartest aren't the best at surviving; those who can adapt to changing circumstances are.

41. Play sports, not (only) for the sake of looking good, but feeling good as well.

42. Embrace constructive criticism and feedback.

43. Keep yourself away from people who bring you down.

44. Relaxing doesn't mean you stopped moving. Healthy breaks are part of the flow.

45. You are not your job. Your career is not your identity. It is what you do. Your spouse and children are not your life — they complement it to perfection.

46. Practice what you preach.

47. Green is good: eat more green food, drink green tea, go out in a green environment, and cross the street only when the light is green for you.

48. Stay true to your beliefs. Don't change them for anybody's sake, just your own.

49. Eat walnuts. They look like a brain for a reason.

50. Print these 50 life-improving steps and read them each morning.

Chapter 7: Final Thoughts

If you've reached this point, it means that you've become richer with lots of tips and tactics regarding your daily routines and habits. You have new weapons to use to defeat procrastination, become more productive, and develop new daily routines based on new perspectives from alternative philosophies. Now you just have to practice. Find your place in the big picture. Some good tips can always expand the possibilities.

If you want to organize an area of your life, prioritize first. When that's done, start working on it. Deal with one to three things at a time. Do not divide your attention and energy. Learn the new mechanisms, and when you can apply them well before you move on, then take on one to three new habits.

1. **Focus on what you want**. Many people concentrate on what they want to avoid. They do not want to be overweight anymore. They do not want to cause an accident. Focus on what you want, not what you don't want. Know where you are now and where you are heading.

2. **Make your goal irresistible**. Don't just say to yourself, "*Yep, I want to be slim, strong, energetic, and rich...*" Instead, use something like: "*I want to burst with energy. I will be more active, I will be stronger, and I will be an example to my kids/my family/my friends*." You need to envision your goal so clearly that it makes you take the first steps. Create an image

that pulls you toward it. Make the goal so irresistible that you immediately want to get started reaching it and developing that particular area.

Your quality of life will improve because you are excited about where you are headed. Your adrenaline level will increase suddenly, and that's a good feeling.

3. **Find the best tools**. Find the path to reaching your goal and solving the problem. If it doesn't exist, you have to build it. Find the starting point. Create it, if there isn't one. It is great if you are enthusiastic and focused. However, it doesn't matter how focused you are and what you believe in if you are using the wrong tools. The wrong strategy or an inappropriate map won't get you closer to your goal, either.

You can find good tools if you imitate someone who is successful at something you want to be successful at. If you emulate someone, you can save time, energy, and money. If you know someone with outstanding results who is already successful, why would you want to reinvent the wheel?

Success always leaves lasting traces. Find the very best in your field, see what they do and how they do it, and copy them. Develop your own style and monitor the process. Adjust what is already working instead of conducting time-consuming experiments.

4. **Break up your inner conflicts**, which often lead to the death of action.

Several forces are fighting with each other when there is an internal conflict. You are the one who can use these forces to your benefit. Inner conflicts are often caused by the lack of knowing "why." Why do you want what you want? Why do you want that particular goal?

You might think that being successful and making a lot of money is immoral, not spiritual. Maybe you want to be spiritual, and in light of this you get in the way of your own financial success.

How can we resolve these inner conflicts and unleash the power of their forces? There is only one way: identify the most important thing for you to do today.

Do not make a decision based on what others expect you to do, or what happened in your past. What your parents, friends, or society wants is irrelevant. When you identify the conflict, bring the values you represent into harmony with your life. Be in agreement with the things that are most important to you.

You will see, once you are in harmony and resolve your inner conflict, that action will take place almost by itself. Be open and accept the incredibly gratifying experience of the "aha" moment. Once you spiritually catch up to your desires and take action, what will happen?

You will reach your goal. Do not stop there. Pass your knowledge on. Help others. Show others what you have and what you have learned. When you teach others, you share your contentment and the joy that comes with success.

When you reach a goal, practice gratitude. Be grateful for the fact that the remaining hours of today represent eternity. Be grateful for being lucky, as these hours are priceless gifts. Be thankful for being able to reach the goal you wanted. This gives us a great advantage over those who thanked yesterday for their lives and are no longer among us today.

You have the chance to become the person you want to be. You only have one life, and think of it as a unit of time. Think about your life. If you are wasting your time procrastinating, you destroy your life. Maximize the use of every hour because you know you can't ever get those hours back. You cannot put them in a bank account to use one day. A dying man would give all his money to have more breaths.

How do you value the hours you have? Make them priceless!

Take care of today's tasks today. Learn to see the joy in things. Remember, you can be as happy as you allow yourself to be.

I believe in you!

Yours truly,

Zoe

Reference

Andrade, Jackie. What does doodling do? University of Plymouth. 2010. https://pearl.plymouth.ac.uk/bitstream/handle /10026.1/4701/Andrade_Doodling%20author %20version.pdf?sequence=1

Bergland, Cristopher. Exposure to Natural Light Improves Workplace Performance. Psychology Today. 2013. www.psychologytoday.com/blog/the-athletes-way/201306/exposure-natural-light-improves-worklace-performance

Christopher M. Jung., Sat Bir S. Khalsa., Frank A. J. L. Scheer, Christian Cajochen, Steven W. Lockley, Charles A. Czeisler, Kenneth P. Wright, Jr. Acute Effects of Bright Light Exposure on Cortisol Levels. NCBI. 2013.

https://www.ncbi.nlm.nih.gov/pmc/articles/PMC3686562/

Csikszentmihaly, Mihaly. Flow. HarperCollins e-books. 2008.

Derbyshire, David. Chewing gum boosts brain's performance. Telegraph. 2002. http://www.telegraph.co.uk/news/uknews/1387660/Chewing-gum-boosts-brains-performance.html

Greenhouse Product News. Texas A&M Study Shows Flowers Increase Workplace Creativity. Greenhouse Product News. 2003. https://gpnmag.com/news/texas-am-study-shows-flowers-increase-workplace-creativity/

Irvine, William, B. A Guide to the Good Life: The Ancient Art of Stoic Joy. Oxford University Press. 2008.

Lee, Kate, E., Williams, Kathryn J.H. Sargentc, Leisa D., Williams, Nicholas S.G. Johnson, Katherine A. 40-second green roof views sustain attention: The role of micro-breaks in attention restoration. Science Direct. 2015. https://www.sciencedirect.com/science/article/pii/S0272494415000328

Leroy, Sophie. Why is it so hard to do my work? The challenge of attention residue when switching between work tasks. Science Direct. 2009. https://www.sciencedirect.com/science/article/pii/S0749597809000399

MacLean, Katherine A. Emilio Ferrer, Stephen R. Aichele, David A. Bridwell, Anthony P. Zanesco, Tonya L. Jacobs, Brandon G. King, Erika L. Rosenberg, Baljinder K. Sahdra, Phillip R. Shaver, B. Alan Wallace, George R. Mangun, Clifford D. Saron. Intensive Meditation Training Improves Perceptual Discrimination and Sustained Attention. Sage Journals. 2010. http://journals.sagepub.com/doi/abs/10.1177/0956797610371339

Nass, Clifford. What is multitasking? PBS. 2010. https://www.pbs.org/wgbh/pages/frontline/digitalnation/interviews/nass.html

Newport, Cal. Deep Work. Grand Central Publishing. 2016.

Newport, Cal. So Good They Can't Ignore You. Piatkus Publisher. 2016.

Nittono H., Fukushima M., Yano A., Moriya H. The Power of Kawaii: Viewing Cute Images Promotes a Careful Behavior and Narrows Attentional Focus. NCBI. 2012. https://www.ncbi.nlm.nih.gov/pubmed/23050022

Onyper., Carr, T.L., Farrar, J.S., Floyd, B.R. Cognitive advantages of chewing gum. Now you see them, now you don't. NCBI. 2011. www.ncbi.nlm.nih.gov/pubmed/21645566

Plant Culture Inc. Why Green? Plant Culture Inc. 2016. http://www.plantcultureinc.com/whygreen.ht ml

Rugg, Michael., Andrews, Mark A. W. How does background noise affect our concentration? Scientific American. 2010. https://www.scientificamerican.com/article/ask-the-brains-background-noise/

Scientific American. Gum Chewing May Improve Concentration. Scientific American. 2013. https://www.scientificamerican.com/podcast/episode/gum-chewing-may-improve-concentrati-13-03-26/

Skills You Need. Neuro-Linguistic Programming (NLP). Skills You Need. 2017. https://www.skillsyouneed.com/ps/nlp.html

Verma, Nitun. Dr. Sleep Medicine. Health Grades. 2018.

https://www.healthgrades.com/physician/dr-nitun-verma-257gy

Endnotes

_i Verma, Nitun. Dr. *Sleep Medicine*. Health Grades. 2018. https://www.healthgrades.com/physician/dr-nitun-verma-257gy

_{ii} Greenhouse Product News. *Texas A&M Study Shows Flowers Increase Workplace Creativity.* Greenhouse Product News. 2003. https://gpnmag.com/news/texas-am-study-shows-flowers-increase-workplace-creativity/

_{iii} Skills You Need. *Neuro-Linguistic Programming (NLP).* Skills You Need. 2017. https://www.skillsyouneed.com/ps/nlp.html

_{iv} Newport, Cal. *So Good They Can't Ignore You*. Piatkus Publisher. 2016.

_v Newport, Cal. *So Good They Can't Ignore You*. Piatkus Publisher. 2016.

_{vi} Irvine, William, B. *A Guide to the Good Life: The Ancient Art of Stoic Joy*. Oxford University Press. 2008.

[vii] Scientific American. *Gum Chewing May Improve Concentration*. Scientific American. 2013. https://www.scientificamerican.com/podcast/episode/gum-chewing-may-improve-concentrati-13-03-26/

[viii] Derbyshire, David. *Chewing gum boosts brain's performance*. Telegraph. 2002. http://www.telegraph.co.uk/news/uknews/1387660/Chewing-gum-boosts-brains-performance.html

[ix] Onyper., Carr, T.L., Farrar, J.S., Floyd, B.R. *Cognitive advantages of chewing gum. Now you see them, now you don't*. NCBI. 2011. www.ncbi.nlm.nih.gov/pubmed/21645566

[x] Rugg, Michael., Andrews, Mark A. W. *How does background noise affect our concentration?* Scientific American. 2010. https://www.scientificamerican.com/article/ask-the-brains-background-noise/

[xi] MacLean, Katherine A. Emilio Ferrer, Stephen R. Aichele, David A. Bridwell, Anthony P. Zanesco, Tonya L. Jacobs, Brandon G. King, Erika L. Rosenberg, Baljinder K. Sahdra, Phillip R. Shaver, B. Alan Wallace, George R. Mangun, Clifford D. Saron. *Intensive Meditation Training Improves Perceptual Discrimination and Sustained Attention.* Sage Journals. 2010. http://journals.sagepub.com/doi/abs/10.1177/0956797610371339

xii Andrade, Jackie. *What does doodling do?* University of Plymouth. 2010. https://pearl.plymouth.ac.uk/bitstream/handle/10026.1/4701/Andrade_Doodling%20author%20version.pdf?sequence=1

xiii Lee, Kate, E., Williams, Kathryn J.H. Sargentc, Leisa D., Williams, Nicholas S.G. Johnson, Katherine A. *40-second green roof views sustain attention: The role of micro-breaks in attention restoration.* Science Direct. 2015. https://www.sciencedirect.com/science/article/pii/S0272494415000328

xiv Bergland, Cristopher. *Exposure to Natural Light Improves Workplace Performance.* Psychology Today. 2013. www.psychologytoday.com/blog/the-athletes-way/201306/exposure-natural-light-improves-worklace-performance

xv Christopher M. Jung., Sat Bir S. Khalsa., Frank A. J. L. Scheer, Christian Cajochen, Steven W. Lockley, Charles A. Czeisler, Kenneth P. Wright, Jr. *Acute Effects of Bright Light Exposure on Cortisol Levels.* NCBI. 2013. https://www.ncbi.nlm.nih.gov/pmc/articles/PMC3686562/

xvi Plant Culture Inc. *Why Green?* Plant Culture Inc. 2016. http://www.plantcultureinc.com/whygreen.html

xvii Nittono H., Fukushima M., Yano A., Moriya H. *The Power of Kawaii: Viewing Cute Images*

Promotes a Careful Behavior and Narrows Attentional Focus. NCBI. 2012.
https://www.ncbi.nlm.nih.gov/pubmed/23050022

[xviii] Leroy, Sophie. *Why is it so hard to do my work? The challenge of attention residue when switching between work tasks.* Science Direct. 2009.
https://www.sciencedirect.com/science/article/pii/S0749597809000399

[xix] Nass, Clifford. *What is multitasking?* PBS. 2010.
https://www.pbs.org/wgbh/pages/frontline/digitalnation/interviews/nass.html

[xx] Csikszentmihaly, Mihaly. *Flow.* HarperCollins e-books. 2008.

[xxi] Newport, Cal. *Deep Work.* Grand Central Publishing. 2016.

88617073R00112

Made in the USA
Columbia, SC
01 February 2018